18 YOGA F[ ]
FOR
TIGHT HAMSTRINGS

BY MĂDĂLINA CIORBA

Website: https://www.yogawithmadalina.com
Instagram: https://instagram.com/yogawithmadalina
TikTok: https://tiktok.com/@yogawithmadalina

The best way to stay up-to-date is to join the email list.
Visit www.yogawithmadalina.com

TABLE OF CONTENTS

INTRODUCTION

First of all thank you for purchasing this book and starting your own yoga journey. It's going to be an exciting experience with lots of great achievements.

The benefits of yoga practice are universal. Yoga attracts people from various ages, socioeconomic levels, ethnicities, and religions. Some have physical restrictions or injuries, while others are in excellent health. So in conclusion anyone can do yoga.

The hamstrings are located in the back of our thighs, and are a group of three long muscles: biceps femoris, semimembranosus and semitendinosus. They originate from the sit bones (ischial tuberosity) and are inserted in the shinbone (tibia) and calf bone (fibula).

You're maybe asking yourself if you have tight hamstrings. Let's see some of the symptoms:
- Lower back pain and stiffness
- Knee pain
- Pain that radiates in the buttocks and back of the leg (also known as sciatica pain)
- You can't touch your toes while your knees are locked
- If you can't straighten your legs completely
- Bad posture
- Imbalance in the muscles

If you cross one or more from this list... I'm sorry to say but you have tight hamstrings.

The main causes of tightness in the hamstring area are: prolonged sitting down (desk job, lifestyle), never stretching your muscles, and sciatic nerve problems. It can also be genetic, but we're talking now about the above.

When our three hamstring muscles are shortened, our pelvis will gain a posterior tilt, flattening our lower back's natural curve and causing our hip flexors to get tight and prone to injury and pain.

You also have to strengthen your core muscles and quadriceps to prevent injury. But you must also include stretching and foam rolling.

Now here is my favorite part: yoga poses that help us stretch our hamstring muscles and keep us pain- and injury-free.

But before we start our yoga practice, I need you to consult your physician if you have any injuries, surgeries, or other illnesses (high blood pressure, glaucoma, etc.) so you won't hurt yourself and cause more pain or damage.

After you've gotten the "ok" from your doctor, we're ready to start.

And I must say this: the stretches should not cause you excruciating pain; that means you're pushing yourself too hard. It should feel good with a little bit of tension but pain-free. Be patient with yourself and your body.

To begin your yoga journey, you won't need fancy equipment or a flexible body. You just need to start here, now, wherever you are. For more comfort, when doing the floor poses, I suggest using a yoga mat or doing them on a carpeted floor. You can find yoga mats almost everywhere and for cheap; just be sure they are not very slippery. As for yoga blocks and straps (belts), you can get them for extra help with the poses. Or you can get creative and use some books and blankets as blocks—just make sure they are stable—and a bathrobe or dress belt or a leather belt for the yoga strap.

ABOUT THE AUTHOR

My name is Mădălina Ciorba and I absolutely adore yoga! I like to keep myself busy and moving by taking part in a variety of activities. After sustaining a back injury, I started practicing yoga frequently.

I used to play tennis, go to the gym, lift weights, do Pilates, run, roller skate, and participate in all sorts of outdoor activities. Until one terrible day, when I suddenly felt a sharp and excruciating pain in my lower back, bringing me to my knees. I couldn't breathe or move! The funny thing is, I got the pain when I was doing some easy and gentle warmup exercises!

The pain lasted a couple of days, and no painkiller could tone it down a notch; I couldn't walk or sit, and there was no way to bend or get up. Because my back hurt so much, laughing or sneezing were my worst nightmares.

After a few days, I finally went to the doctor and got an MRI. The diagnosis was Discopathy... Two of my lumbar intervertebral discs were damaged. And the doctor said I couldn't play any more sports that included sudden moves, twists, or any pressure on my lower spine. That, for me, was horrifying! No more tennis, gym, running, or anything fun—not even pilates or jumping!

My world got a massive shake. The things I really enjoyed and that kept me active were no longer within my reach. I felt a bit lost and overwhelmed. Then I asked myself, "Now what?"

I tried to take things more easily and started with some kinesiotherapy and laser treatments. After a few sessions, I started to feel much better. But it was not enough; I really missed playing sports and being active. As I was doing my medical gymnastics exercises, I started to notice that some of them actually resembled yoga poses. I asked my therapist if I could maybe start doing yoga. She said I could only do gentle exercises that don't put any stress on my lower back.

Gradually incorporating a few gentle yoga exercises into my daily routine made me discover the long-forgotten passion for yoga I'd gotten from my first teacher a few years ago. She inspired my journey toward discovering my passion for yoga.

I started to slowly increase the difficulty of the exercises and their duration, which made me feel much better and, best of all, made the pain disappear completely.

I couldn't believe it! Yoga helped me recover from my injury and brought back some of the other activities I used to do, like roller skating and running.

After a few months, I was almost back to my old self, but I was a bit more careful with my back, which meant no more carrying or lifting heavy stuff.

I started to attend different yoga classes. I was glad to return to the sweet pain of muscle soreness and not back pain.

As I attended more classes and caught the "yoga bug", I began to consider becoming a yoga teacher in the back of my mind.

After a quick search for "Yoga Teacher Trainings" near me, I found one that was relatively close to my town and began in the spring.

Because of my back discomfort, moderate to poor flexibility, and the fact that I had never taught anything to anyone before, I was skeptical that I would be able to complete the 200-hour program.

But, in the end, I chose to face my fears and apply for the TTC. I was both excited and nervous to begin.

A lot happened in the few months before the training course began. I just married the love of my life, and it was the year of fresh starts.

Finally the start date of the training program was almost here and I was extremely excited!

Those annoying little doubts and questions started coming out more and more: "What if you are not flexible enough?", "Am I too old for this?", "Are you sure you can teach people? You are not good at public speaking!", "You are going to embarrass yourself!", "Can you even do more intense yoga with your injuries?", "What if you can't learn? It's been a while since you studied!".

Luckily, I have a very supportive husband who helped me through all my intrusive thoughts, doubts, and low self-confidence. That made me feel better about this whole situation.

The "200-hour Teacher Training Course" was challenging and packed with useful new information. I began to understand more about yoga than I had previously.

I've met so many amazing women who were strong, caring, and supportive of one another. The time spent together was so special and magical, and I was quite sad when the training concluded and everyone went their separate ways. I still keep in touch with some of them.

After I completed the training and received my certification, I was proud and blown away. I really did it! I faced all of my fears, doubts and felt like I could do anything.

My body was feeling better than before. It was the middle of summer, and I was pain-free. No more spine discomfort!

I've kept my personal practice since the training, and it sure helped me stay pain-free. In addition, my overall flexibility and mobility increased. Perseverance is the key to a peaceful mind and a healthy body.

I have learned that hamstring stiffness is a component of back pain, so I urge you to check your hamstring flexibility.

In autumn, I started working on another dream project: opening my own yoga studio in my hometown! It was a great deal of work and fun, but I finally found the perfect place to start my yoga studio.

POSE GUIDE

In this book you will find 18 yoga poses (asanas) that help you stretch your tight hamstring muscles, and improve your flexibility.

If you really want to improve your flexibility and practice, I advise you to work on each posture for how many days you need to until you feel like you've "got there". Each body is different, so take it at your own pace, and don't push yourself too hard to avoid injuries.

You might stumble across postures in this book that you have already practiced but whose names vary from those in the book. When new yoga styles are formed and sold, people frequently strive to come up with new English names for the poses in order to distinguish them. You don't need to try to recall the names; they are simply helpful in identifying the postures. The posture's Sanskrit name is also always provided. Nearly all of the positions end with "-asana" which means "posture" or "pose" in Sanskrit.

In the guide below, each pose is accompanied by its unique benefits and step by step instructions on how to enter it. The benefits are articulated to help you understand the impact on your overall health. Each pose has variations of difficulty so you can adjust it to your own level.

You can get creative with the order in which you do the poses. You can start with just 15 minutes of practice and, with time, increase your practice duration and how long you're holding each pose.

Let's get to the fun part: your first asana for improving your hamstring flexibility.

STANDING FORWARD FOLD

UTTANASANA

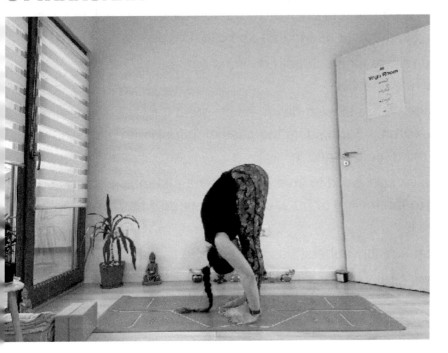

Benefits

- Improves flexibility, it's part of the Sun salutation and vinyasa transitions
- It can be adapted for all levels just by going into the fold less deeply
- Stretches the whole back of your body, including back muscles, buttocks, hamstrings (thighs) and calf muscles
- Helps relieve stomach pain during menstrual periods and improves digestion
- Heartbeats are slowed down, so it's great for people who are overexcited. After holding the pose, you feel calm and cool, and your mind feels at peace
- Helps you get used to inversions like headstands, getting you used to the feeling of pressure in your head when the heart is above it
- We can identify imbalances between the two sides of the body
- Lowers stress and tension in the body

How to

1. Begin by standing with your feet hip-width apart and parallel. Inhale, raise the arms up, and look up. Then exhale, slowly lowering your torso towards your thighs. Hands are reaching for the floor or feet. The lower back must be kept straight.
2. The quadriceps are engaged to straighten the knees, and the hamstrings are stretching.
3. We slightly tilt our pelvis forward.

4. And we bring our chest towards the thighs, or we intend to.

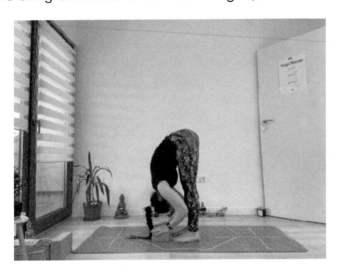

Forward Fold With Yoga Block

5. If our hamstrings are really tight and we have trouble straightening the knees, we might keep a microbend in the knees. And in time, we will work on straightening the legs.

6. Another variation of this pose is a half-forward fold. We bend forward and place our hands on our thighs or shins. And we lengthen the back, keeping it straight and bringing the crown of the head forward. If this is easy, we can try this variation without the hands on our thighs, but keeping them towards the floor or straight ahead.

7. It is important to feel an intense stretch on our back legs, but it shouldn't hurt.

8. When we exit out of the pose, we slowly come up, vertebrae with vertebrae. We can also bend the knees when coming up if we

have lower back pain or injuries. Another way is by placing our hands on our hips and slowly rolling up.

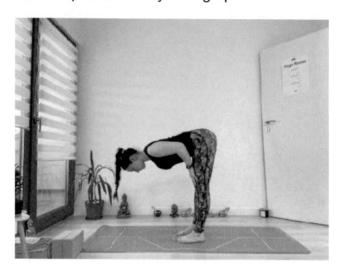

Half Forward Fold

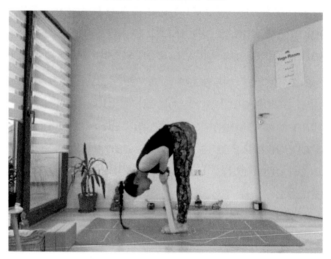

Forward Fold With Yoga Strap

9. You can use some props. A block or a yoga strap. You can place the yoga block in front of you so you can rest your hands on it. You can slowly pull yourself closer to your legs by placing the yoga strap under your feet and using the ends to pull gently.

TRIANGLE POSE

UTTHITA TRIKONASANA

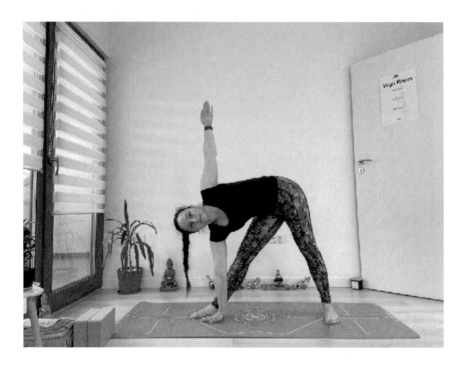

Benefits

- Improves your balance and flexibility
- Reduces nervousness and depression
- Tones and stretches the whole body and helps us overcome weakness in the legs
- Helps us open the hips and groins
- It's helpful in scoliosis and neck strains
- Intense stretch to the sides of the torso and hamstrings

How to

1. We start by standing with our feet hip-width apart. Then we take our right foot and take a big step towards the back of the mat, so we are facing sideways.
2. The distance between our feet should be approx. 120–150 cm (about 4-5 feet), depending on the length of our torso and flexibility. The right foot's heel is placed on the same line as the left foot's arch. Beginners can place the right heel on the left big toe.
3. The arms are spread sideways, palms facing down, parallel with the floor. They should be in line with our shoulders.
4. Next, we should stretch the right arm to the right side (back of the mat), like something is pulling on our arm towards them or like we want to reach something.
5. Then slowly go down, with the right hand reaching towards the outer side of the right foot. If we can't go that low without

compromising our shape, we can reach for our shin or the top of the foot.

6. We can use props like a yoga block here. Place the block on the outer side of the foot and place your hand on it.
7. Now stretch your left arm towards the ceiling, keeping it in line with your shoulders. The arms should now be forming a straight line.
8. Now we switch feet and repeat for the other side.

Tips

✦ We should bring our front knee towards the little toe, externally rotating our leg.

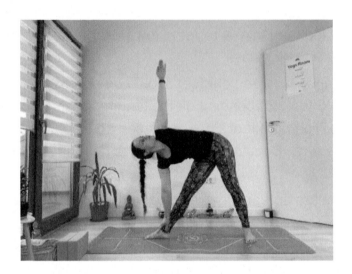

Triangle With Hand on Leg

✦ Our back and hips should be in line with the back of our legs. Knee in line with the shoulder.

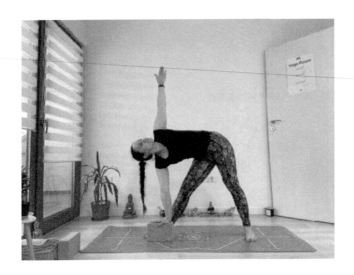

Triangle With Yoga Block

✦ We can use the different sides of the yoga block to adjust height.

PYRAMID POSE

PARSVOTTANASANA

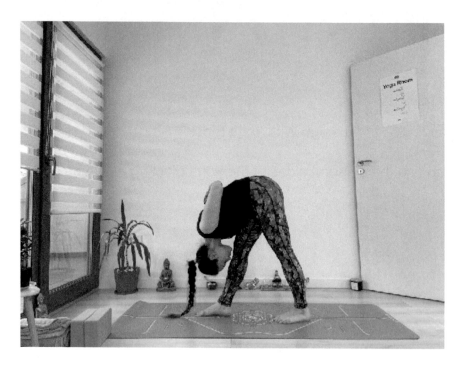

Benefits

- Helps us unlock our hip joints, bringing more mobility
- This pose helps us work deeper on the hamstrings, giving them a good stretch
- Improves digestion by helping the colon work properly
- Tones the abdominal muscles
- Strengthens the quads, calf muscles, ankles, and spine
- Builds support for the lower back

Precautions

- Do not go all the way down if you have a hamstring tear, high blood pressure, or back injuries. You should do only the half-way fold, keeping the torso parallel to the ground.
- If you have suffered a hip injury, you should avoid this pose until you fully recover.

How to

1. Start from standing, then step your right foot back flat on the ground. The distance between the legs should be 1 meter (3–4 feet) or more.
2. Now line up your left heel with the right one. Both feet are pointed towards the front of the mat.
3. We start placing our hands together behind the back, fingers towards the ground, thumbs touching your spine. Now we move our hands so the fingers touch the back. Slowly, we rotate the

hands so the fingers point upwards and slide them up your spine. The shoulders are drawn back, and the chest is expanded.

4. Slowly lift your chest, then fold from your front hip. The torso should rest on the front leg's thigh.
5. The hips must be square, and the thighs must be engaged.
6. Lengthen the spine and try to slightly arch your lower back instead of rounding your entire back.
7. Now straighten your legs by engaging your quads, but don't hyperextend your knees. Keep the legs strong and feel the stretch in the hamstrings and calves.
8. To come out, slowly lift your torso while keeping your legs straight. If that is too hard, you can bend the front knee.
9. Now repeat on the other side.

Variations

✦ If reverse prayer hands are too difficult, you can simply grab the opposite elbow. Or you can grab the wrists.
✦ Another way is to place the hands on the floor on each side of the front foot. If you can't reach the floor, you can place yoga blocks under your hands.
✦ If you find it difficult to fold all the way down, you can go down just halfway with the half pyramid pose. Or you can use a chair or wall to hold on to while bending halfway.

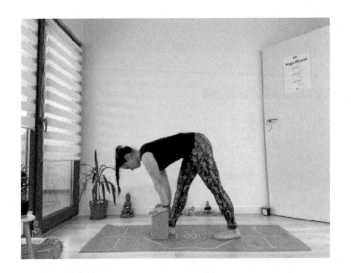

Half Pyramid With Yoga Blocks

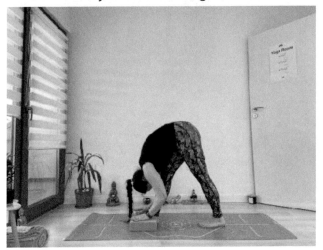

Pyramid With Yoga Blocks

WARRIOR I

VIRABHADRASANA I

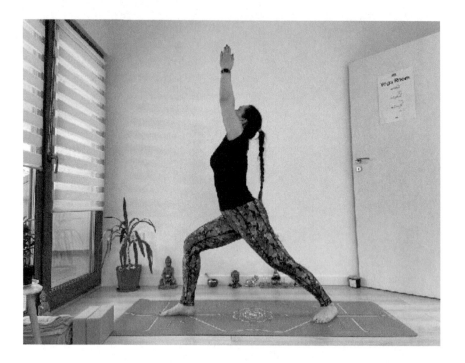

Benefits

- Improves focus and balance by getting us to engage our deep core muscles
- Helps strengthen the arms, shoulders, legs, and back muscles
- This pose is a chest and hip opener
- It gives us a nice stretch of the psoas, quads, and back leg muscles
- Can help with sciatica pain
- Stabilize the knee joint by strengthening the muscles around it
- By opening our chests, we encourage deep breathing

Precautions

- It is very important to talk to your physician before doing this pose if you have any hip surgery or replacement, hamstring tears, or spine issues.

How to

1. Start from standing, feet hip-width apart, with arms and shoulders relaxed. Step your left foot back, turning your toes at a 45-degree angle. The distance between feet should be about 60 to 100 cm (approximately 2–3 feet).
2. The right foot's toes are pointing toward the front. Heels should be on the same line. If you find it difficult to balance, you can keep your heels on two parallel lines, slightly wider.
3. Bend the front right knee at a 90-degree angle, making sure the shin is perpendicular to the mat and the thigh is almost parallel to

the floor. Keep your knee stacked over the ankle and don't let it collapse inward. Straighten your left knee by engaging your leg muscles.

4. Bring your torso to face the front leg, making sure your hips are aligned and both pointing forward. Inhale and bring your arms up, palms together facing each other, and lower the shoulders from your ears, creating some space. Keep the chest open, and if you're feeling ready, slowly look up towards the thumbs of your hands, keeping the neck relaxed. Maintain for a few breaths, then change sides.

Variations

✦ Point your tailbone down towards the mat and engage your abdomen to draw your lower belly in. It's important not to put pressure on your lower back.

✦ If your back leg hurts while keeping it straight, you can move forward on the ball of your foot, like in a high lunge. And if it still hurts, you can also bend the knee a bit.

✦ If you feel too much pressure on the lower back and it starts to hurt, shorten the distance between your feet or come more up on the bent leg, making the pose less straining on your lumbar area.

✦ Another variation of the arms can be used if you have very tight shoulders. You can put your hands together in front of your chest in prayer position (Namaste hands) and bring your gaze forward for more balance. Or keep hands up but not together, keeping them at shoulder-width distance.

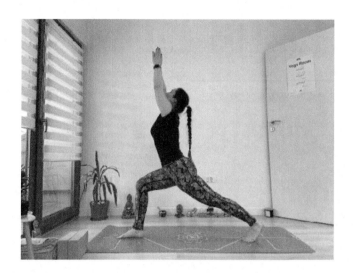

Warrior 1 With Raised Heel

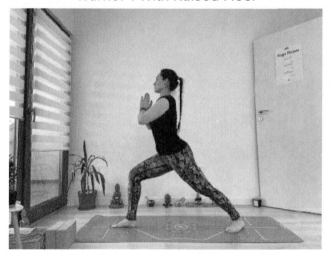

Warrior 1 With Namaste Hands

STANDING WIDE-LEGGED FORWARD FOLD

PRASARITA PADOTTANASANA

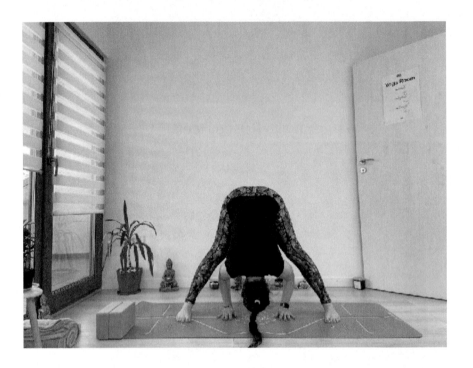

Benefits

- Stretches the hamstrings and the inner thigh muscles (adductors)
- Also a good hip opener and deep hip flexor
- Helps lengthen the spine and neck, releasing tension
- Improves our flexibility and strength
- Reduces back pain caused by stiffness
- Tones the legs

How to

1. Start from standing; feet are hip distance apart; upper body is relaxed.
2. Step your left foot to the back of the mat with a swipe motion, opening the hips to the side.
3. The toes of both feet are pointed to the side of the mat, and the distance between them should be at least 100 cm (3.2 feet) or more, depending on your height and flexibility.
4. Keep the knees as straight as you can without hyper-flexion. Engage your quadriceps to straighten the knees.
5. Inhale and bring the arms parallel to the ground, then place the hands on your hips. With an exhale, start lowering your torso towards the thighs. When going down, keep the lower back as straight as possible, using a pelvic tilt.
6. Stay here for a breath or two, then place the palms on the mat, between the legs (in line with the feet). And try to bring the crown of the head towards the mat, in front of your palms. Place most of your weight on the front part of the foot, on the ball of your feet.

You should feel an intense stretch sensation in the back and inside of the legs.

7. To get up, you can slightly bend your knees and slowly come up halfway, keeping the back straight, then all the way up. Keep the arms parallel to the ground. Then step the left foot back to the front of the mat, turning the toes towards the front of the mat, making your way back to standing. Or you can get creative and turn your torso towards the right leg and place your hands on the mat, stepping the right foot back into Downward Facing Dog.

Variations

+ If your hamstrings are really tight and you can't reach the mat with your hands, you can place yoga blocks so you can rest your palms on them.

+ This pose has some fun variations: you can keep your hands on your hips and bend forward, letting your head hang heavy towards the ground. Another one is interlacing the fingers behind your back so the palms of your hand are facing away from you, then slowly bending forward, letting the palms go heavy towards the mat. This one is a great shoulder stretch, too. And the last one is grabbing the big toes with your index and middle fingers, bending the elbows to 90 degrees, and bringing the head down to the ground.

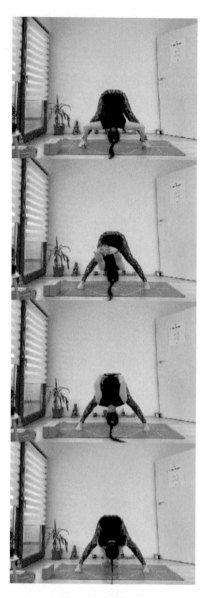

DOWN FACING DOG/DOWNWARD DOG

ARDHO MUKHA SVANASANA

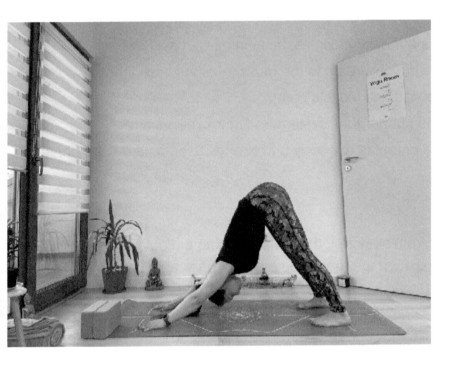

Benefits

- Opens the chest and the shoulders
- Gives us strength in the arms, shoulders, and legs
- Great hip opener
- Tones our back muscles, helping us with posture
- Gives a nice stretch to the muscles of the back legs
- Relieves back muscle pain
- Calms our nervous system and helps relieve stress
- Helps energize our body and is often used as a resting pose

How to

1. Start from standing, then fold, bringing the palms to the mat on each side of the feet. Step one foot back and then the other in a high plank.
2. Now bring your sitting bones up towards the ceiling and back, pressing through the palms and fingers. The fingers are spread wide on the mat, the hands and feet are shoulder-width apart. The weight is distributed evenly between the legs and palms.
3. Slowly straighten the legs, trying to gently push your heels towards the ground.
4. Shoulders are kept away from your ears by bringing the shoulder blades down on your back and apart.
5. Push your chest towards your thighs, keeping your gaze towards your pelvis or legs. The lower back and spine should be as straight as possible. Maintain the tailbone in a neutral position.

6. Hold the pose for a few breaths.

Variations

✦ For really tight hamstrings, you can keep the knees a little bent and try to peddle the feet to loosen the muscles. Or place a folded blanket under your heels for more support.

✦ This pose is a well-known one, and it's used in Sun Salutation (Surya Namaskar), transitioning, and vinyasa. It's also used as a resting position. There are a few ways to enter Downward Facing Dog. The first way is described in the How to above.

✦ The second way to enter this pose is from Tabletop, where your knees are stacked under the hips and your wrists under the shoulders. Curl your toes under and slowly push your sitting bones up and back. Adjust the distance between hands and feet as needed.

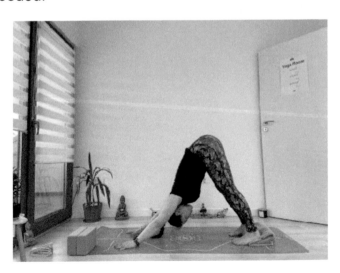

Downward Dog With Folded Blanket

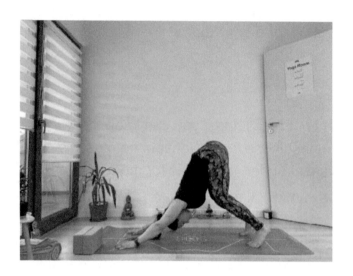

Downward Dog With Bent Knees

✦ Another way is from Upward Dog, when you do a vinyasa or a transition. Again, curl the toes (or roll on the toes) and bring the hips up and back. You can also find your own creative way to get into Downward Facing Dog.

STANDING SPLIT

URDHVA PRASARITA EKA PADASANA

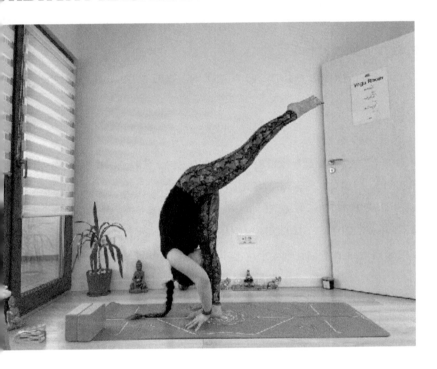

Benefits

- Helps bring more flexibility to the hips and spine
- Makes the spine and legs more strong
- Improves the function of the kidneys and liver
- Gives a good stretch to the hamstrings, quads, and calves
- Increases the blood flow and improves our breathing
- Helps with your balance
- This pose also helps calm the mind, so you can concentrate

How to

1. Start from Downward Facing Dog and step the right sole between your palms. Transfer your weight to the right leg and slowly lift the left leg, keeping your palms on the mat. You can place your palms in front of the standing leg.

2. Lift the left leg up towards the ceiling, keeping the knee straight and the toes pointed. The right knee is angled to the front, not inward.

3. Hips are staked side by side, not angled to one side. If you can't lift the leg higher, don't open up the hip to the side.

4. Bring the chest toward the standing leg, taking care not to round the lombar spine. Only the upper back can be rounded if you need to. Draw your abdomen towards the spine. Remember to lengthen the spine.

5. Draw the crown of your head down to the mat, keeping the neck relaxed. Now place the hands on your thigh or shin, or keep them on the ground. Hold the pose for a couple of breaths.

6. To exit the pose, remove hands from the right leg, slowly hinge from the hips, release the left leg to the mat, and come to a

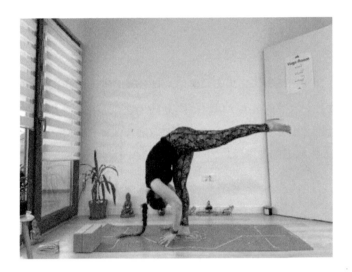

Half Standing Split

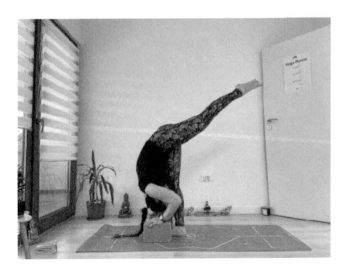

Standing Split With Yoga Blocks

Forward Fold. Then step back to Downward Facing Dog and repeat on the other side.

Variations

- ✦ You can also use the wall to get a deeper stretch.
- ✦ You can bring the leg just half way up, keeping the hands on blocks. Be careful not to overstretch your hamstrings. Keep a microbend in the standing leg knee.

HALF SPLIT

ARDHA HANUMANASANA

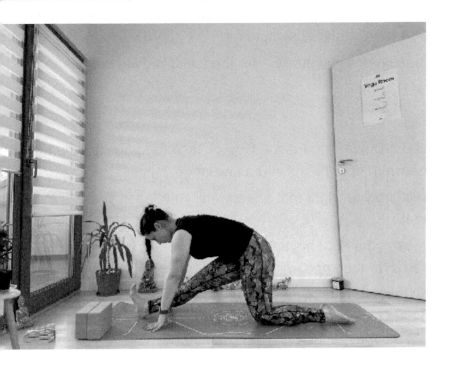

Benefits

- Intense stretch to the hip area and hamstrings, increasing the range of motion
- Increases blood flow in the groin area
- Helps you get more patient, reducing anxiety and stress levels
- Gentle stretch to the lower back, ankles, and soles, helping ease plantar fasciitis-related symptoms
- This pose helps you prepare for the full split (Hanumanasana)

How to

1. Start from Downward Facing Dog or Tabletop and step the right foot between your palms into a low lunge.
2. Start sliding your right foot ahead until your leg is straight and on the heel.
3. Now push your right hip back so the hips are in line. Keep the hip stacked over the knee.
4. Slowly bring the hands further up beside the right leg until your chest gets closer to the right thigh. Try to keep your back as straight as you can and tilt your pelvis forward. You should feel an intense stretch in your right hamstring, calf, and glute.
5. Hold the pose for a couple of breaths then come back to Downward Facing Dog and then low lunge, changing the side.

Variations

- If you can't reach the mat with your hands and you have to flex your thoracic spine, it's better to place some blocks under the palms to keep the back as straight as you can.
- Or you can use a yoga strap if you can't reach your foot at all, placing it on the sole of your foot and holding it with your hands to get the stretch. If your hamstrings are tight, you can always keep a small bend in your front knee.

Precautions

- Precautions should be taken if you suffer a hamstring or lower back injury. It is very important to do a proper warm-up before doing any pose.

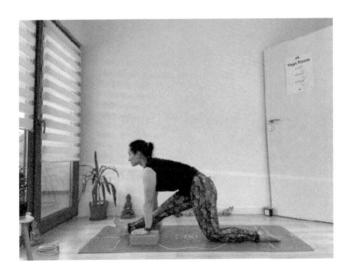

Half Split With Yoga Blocks

LIZARD POSE

UTTHAN PRISTHASANA

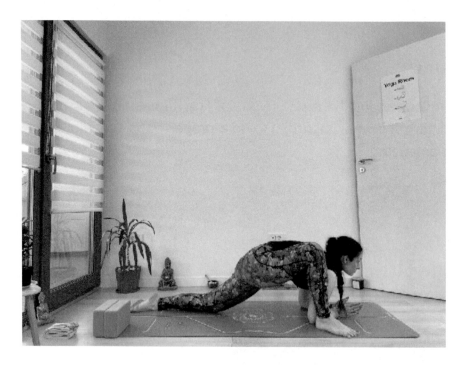

Benefits

- This pose helps us both mentally and physically by decreasing stress, improving our focus, increasing creativity, and reducing negative emotions
- Stretches the flexor muscles, groin, hamstrings, and quads
- It is an intense hip opener that might surface some emotions that are stored in the hips. It is normal to feel a bit more emotional after working on your hip area
- Improves flexibility in our legs and hips. Strengthens the hamstrings and quads, giving us more stability
- Gives us an energy boost in the body and stimulates the internal organs
- Because it's a deep stretch to the pelvic area, it activates the reproductive system and decreases symptoms related to menopause

How to

1. This pose starts like the previous one, in Downward Facing Dog or Tabletop. Bring your right leg between the palms and let the left knee rest on the mat.
2. Wiggle the sole of the right foot to the side of the mat and turn the toes slightly towards the side, bringing both hands inside the right leg. Keep the knee bent, being careful that the knee doesn't go over the toes and is in line with the ankle.
3. Now push the hips forward, stretching the left quadriceps and opening up the right hip.

4. Slowly lower your torso, getting on the forearms but keeping the back as straight as you can. Your gaze is down or a little bit in front of the palms, keeping the neck relaxed.

5. Push your hips forward and down, feeling an intense stretch sensation in the hips and hamstrings. Keep the hips squared, facing forward, and do not let them twist to the side.

6. Keep your chest open and don't collapse into your shoulders by engaging your core muscles. This also helps you protect your lower back from pain.

7. Stay in the pose for a few breaths, then come back to Downward Facing Dog or Tabletop and change sides.

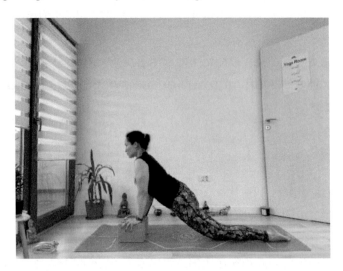

Lizard With Straight Arms And Yoga Blocks

Variations

+ If lowering down makes your back curve, use blocks under the hands or forearms.

✦ You can keep the back knee on the mat or lift it up for a more engaging variation.

Precautions

✦ If you have any knee or hip injuries, it is better to avoid this pose until you recover and then consult a specialist before attempting it. Also, you should be careful if you have weak shoulder joints because this pose puts some pressure on that area.

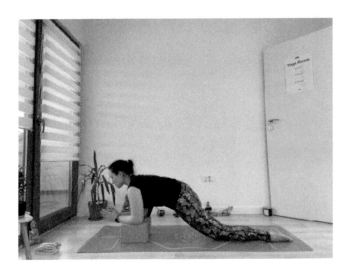

Lizard With Yoga Blocks

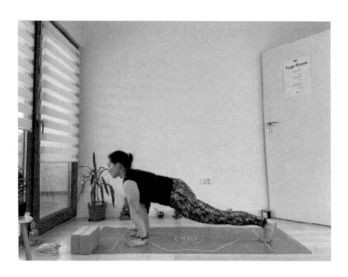

Lizard With Raised Knees

SIDE LUNGE POSE

SKANDASANA

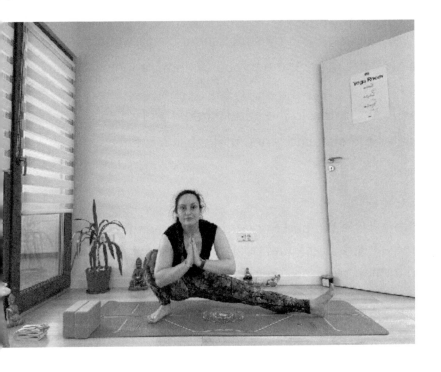

Benefits

◉ Improves flexibility of hips, pelvic area, hamstrings and calves

◉ Strengthens the core, legs, knees, and ankles, bringing more balance to the body and better posture

◉ Gives a good stretch to the hip area, hamstrings, quads, calves, ankles, and soles

◉ Improves our breathing by stretching the intercostal muscles

◉ Helps calm the mind and nervous system, reducing anxiety and stress levels

◉ Improves blood flow to the head, knees, and ankles

◉ Stimulates the circulatory and metabolic systems

How to

1. Start from Wide Legged Forward Fold (Prasarita Padottanasana) and come into a half squat position, keeping your hands on the mat in front of you.

2. Shift your weight to the left side and slowly straighten the right leg to the side by engaging your quad muscles.

3. Bring the toes of the right foot towards you by having only the heel on the mat. Keep the heels on the same line and the toes of the bent leg pointing in the same direction as the knee. The heel of the left foot is on the mat.

4. Shift your hips back, keeping the spine long by using your core muscles, and push the sitting bones towards the mat. Try to keep the left hip open by engaging your inner thigh.

5. When you feel stable enough, slowly bring your hands up, palms together, in front of your chest.
6. Hold the pose for a few breaths, and then come up to Wide Legged Forward Fold and switch legs.

Variations

✦ If you can't bring the heel of the bent leg to the mat, keep the hands on the mat for extra balance, and slowly push the heel towards the mat.

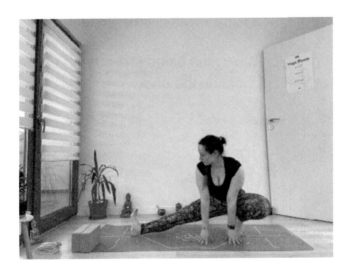

Side Lunge With Raised Heel

Precautions

✦ You shouldn't practice this pose if you have any injuries or surgeries in the hip area, knees, ankles, or spine. Take

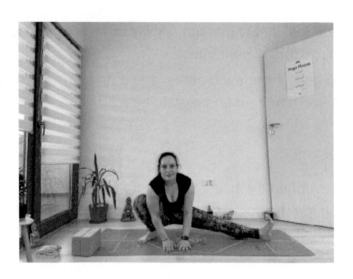

Side Lunge With Hands On Mat

precautions if you have high blood pressure or are recovering from illnesses that weaken the body.

PANCAKE FOLD (WIDE ANGLE SEATED FORWARD FOLD)

UPAVISTHA KONASANA

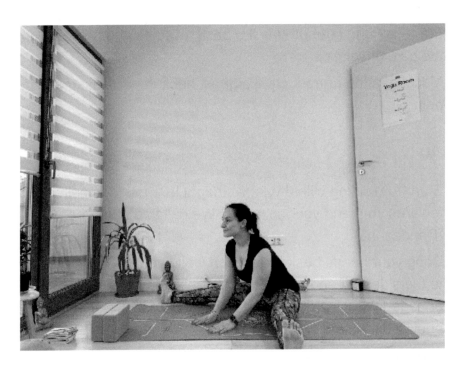

Benefits

- This deep stretch pose has some really amazing mental benefits, reducing stress, anxiety, and mild depression while also soothing the nervous system
- Makes you more flexible by stretching the hips, hamstrings, knees, calves, lower back, abdomen, and shoulders
- Helps relieve digestive issues like indigestion and constipation by enhancing the digestive system
- Stretches and strengthens the back muscles and helps reduce the pain of sciatica
- Massages the reproductive organs, helping decrease menstrual pain

How to

1. Start from sitting with the legs straight in front, toes pointing towards you, and your spine tall. We call this Staff Pose (Dandasana).
2. Bring your hands back for support while you open your legs wide to the sides. Keep the kneecaps pointing up and the leg muscles engaged. Your pelvis is in an anterior tilt, and the spine is kept neutral during the forward fold.
3. Now place the palms in front of you and slowly go forward by hinging from the hips first, and move the hands further away to get the chest closer to the mat. You should feel an intense stretch in the inner thigh and back of the legs, but it shouldn't hurt too much. If you are experiencing intense pain, lift your torso and keep a microbend in your knees.

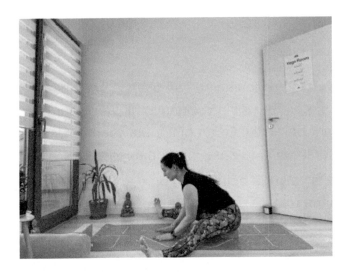

Pancake Fold With Yoga Block

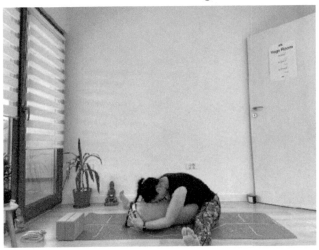

Pancake Fold With Bolster

Variations

- ✦ If you find it too difficult, you can place a yoga block (folded blanket) under your sitting bones to elevate your hips, but keep the anterior pelvic tilt. Or a bolster between the legs so you can rest the torso on it, to ease into the pose and stretch.
- ✦ You can use a yoga belt (strap) on each foot and pull yourself closer to the mat.

Precautions

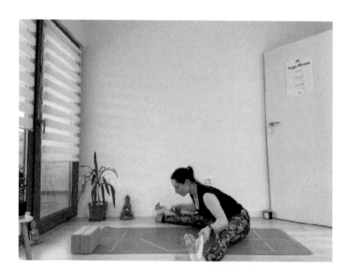

Pancake Fold With Yoga Straps

- ✦ If you have suffered any groin or hamstring tears, you should avoid this pose. And it's important that you consult a professional doctor if you've had a herniated disc or spine surgery.

SITTING FORWARD BEND

PASCHIMOTTANASANA

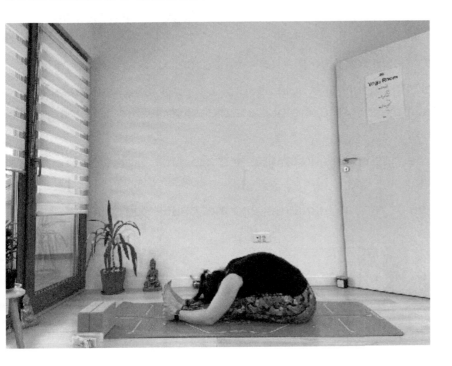

Benefits

- This folding pose helps calm the nervous system, which reduces stress and anxiety.
- Tones the thighs and abdomen area, as well as the reproductive organs
- It mildly decompresses the spine, giving you a little bit more "height"
- It is a deep stretch on the hamstrings, spine, and calves muscles
- By folding deeply and holding it for a longer time, you massage and stimulate your excretory and digestive systems, helping with constipation
- Reduces insomnia and fatigue and alleviates high blood pressure and sinusitis
- Also helps reduce menstrual and menopause discomfort

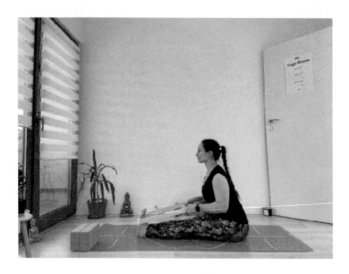

Sitting Forward Bend With Yoga Strap

How to

1. Start from Staff Pose (Dandasana) with your legs stretched out in front of you and your back tall. Tilt your pelvis forward and raise your arms up, then slowly come down, bringing the torso toward your thighs by bending from the hips and not by curving the spine.
2. Keep the back of the knee on the mat by engaging your quads. Pull your toes back towards your torso and slightly rotate your thighs towards the middle. Keep the legs engaged while in the pose.
3. If you can reach, grab your big toes with the index and middle fingers. Slowly pull your chest closer to your thighs by bending your elbows. Try not to curve from the lower back, leading with your chest, not your head, when going down. And keep the spine long by bringing the shoulder blades closer together and opening the chest.
4. Stay here for a few breaths, and then slowly get up by placing your hands by the sides of your legs.

Variations

✦ If you can't reach the toes, wrap a yoga strap around the middle part of the soles and use it to pull yourself forward. But remember to keep the lower back straight. If your hamstrings are really tight, you can use a yoga block or folded blanket under the hips and only bend a little until you feel the stretch. As your muscles get more stretched, you can bend forward a little bit more, and in time, you will be able to place your chest on the thighs.

Precautions

✦ Ask a professional before attempting this pose if you are pregnant, have slipped discs, a hernia, or spondylitis.

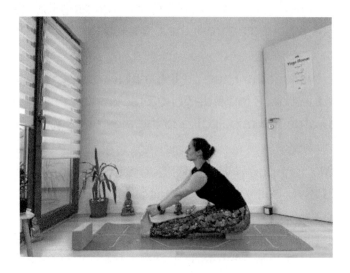

Sitting Forward Bend With Yoga Block

HERON POSE

KROUNCHASANA

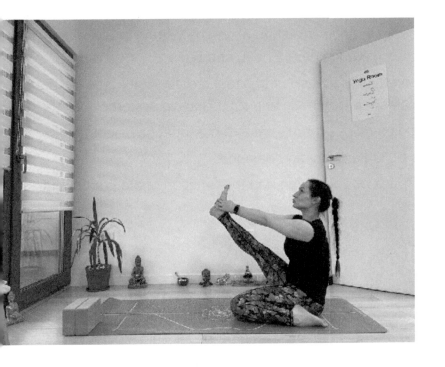

Benefits

- This pose is a little more intermediate, but it helps prepare the body for more advanced practice by improving balance and stability
- As far as mental benefits go, it helps calm the mind, reducing stress and anxiety
- It gives an intense stretch to all the hamstring muscles. And also stretches the shoulders, chest, and back.
- Bringing the leg towards the chest creates compression that stimulates the lymphatic and reproductive systems
- Also helps relieve menstrual and menopause discomfort
- Helps build flexibility and balance
- It improves our digestion and the function of the uterus and ovaries

How to

1. Start from sitting (Dandasana) and bend your left leg, bringing your foot on the outside of your left hip bone. Sit down beside (inside) the bent leg and straighten your right leg in front of you. Both of your sitting bones are on the mat.
2. Sit up tall with your torso and bend your right knee, bringing your heel closer to your sitting bones. Extend both arms down by the sides of your right leg and grab the sole of the foot.
3. Now slowly start straightening your right leg up at an approximately 45-degree angle and lean back a little. Don't round your back; instead, engage your abdominals to keep your spine

long. Try bringing your shoulder blades back to keep your chest open. Bring your foot as high as your head or slightly higher.

4. Hold this pose for a few breaths, then bend the knee and come out of it. Change sides.

Variations

✦ You can modify the pose for a more beginner-friendly option by keeping the left leg straight instead of bent. Then bring the right leg up, but instead of holding your sole, you can hold your ankle or shin. Keep the spine long, and dorsiflex both feet.

✦ Another option is to use a yoga strap on the sole of the raised leg instead of your hands if you can't reach your sole or it's causing you to round your back.

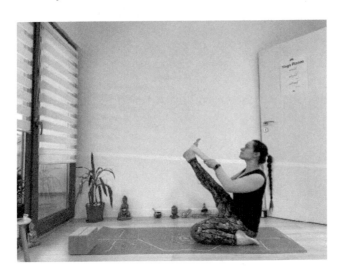

Heron With Yoga Strap

Precautions

✦ This pose is more intermediate to advanced, so you must be really careful when practicing it. It's best if you consult with your physician or specialist before attempting it, especially if you have any knee or ankle issues.

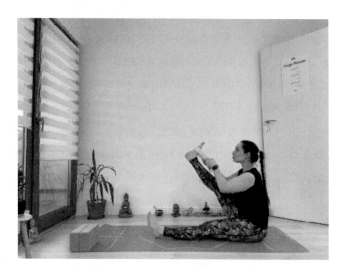

Heron With Straight Leg And Yoga Strap

RECLINED BIG TOE HOLD

SUPTA PADANGUSTHASANA

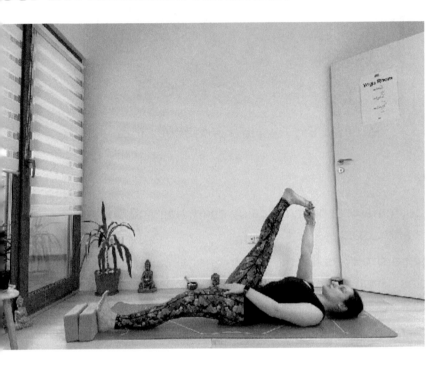

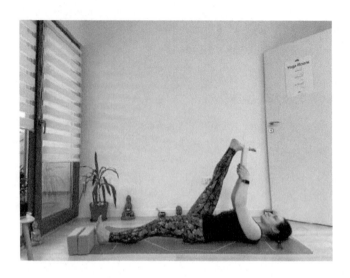

Reclined Big Toe Hold With Yoga Strap

Benefits

- This asymmetrical pose helps us calm the mind and reduce stress and anxiety
- The pose stretches the hips, hamstrings, calves, and psoas muscles. Strengthening the knees and foot arches
- It opens the hips, helping improve mobility and flexibility; it is also a good preparation pose for Hanumanasana (splits)
- Helps relieve sciatica and low back pain
- Keeps our digestion and reproductive health in good condition and helps with menstrual cramps

How to

1. Start from lying down on your back and arching your lower back to push the thighs flat on the mat.

2. Lift the right leg up and bend the knee so you can reach your big toe, going inside the legs. Grab it with your index and middle fingers and straighten the leg, pushing the heel up.

3. Push your left thigh on the mat with the help of your left hand and quads. Remember to keep your shoulders on the mat.

4. Keep the right leg up, letting the back of the leg stretch, and bring it closer to your shoulder or chest.

5. Hold the pose for a couple of breaths. Bring the leg down to the mat and change sides.

ariations

✦ If you find it difficult to keep the leg straight, you can keep a small bend in the right knee. And if you can't reach your toe without bringing your shoulders up from the mat, use a yoga strap placed

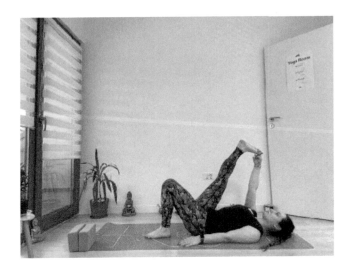

Reclined Big Toe Hold With Bent Leg

on the middle of the sole and grab the ends of the strap to pull your leg towards you.

+ If you're experiencing lower back discomfort, you can keep the other leg, which is on the mat, bent and your sole on the mat so there is less pressure on the lumbar area.

HAPPY BABY POSE

ANANDA BALASANA

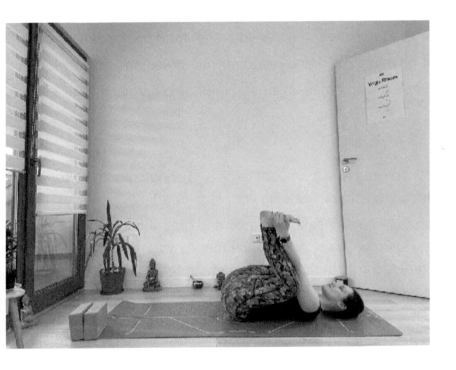

Benefits

- This pose is very good for women who suffer from chronic pelvic pain and also alleviates menstrual cramping
- It massages the abdominal organs, improving kidney function and the blood filtration process by removing toxins from your body
- Realigns the spine and gives you relief from back pain
- Helps calm the mind and reduces your stress and anxiety levels
- Stretches the spine, hips, inner thighs, and hamstrings

How to

1. Start from lying down on your back and bringing both of your knees to your chest, keeping your legs apart.
2. Reach both arms inside your legs and grab the outside of your soles. Push the lower back to the mat as you push the soles of your feet towards the ceiling, flexing the toes and creating some resistance.
3. Keep the knees at a 90-degree angle and the shins perpendicular to the mat, wider than your torso. Bring the knees closer to your armpits. Try keeping the shoulders on the mat and the neck relaxed. Push your tailbone forward and down to create more openness in the sacrum and low back.
4. Hold this pose for a few breaths.

Variations

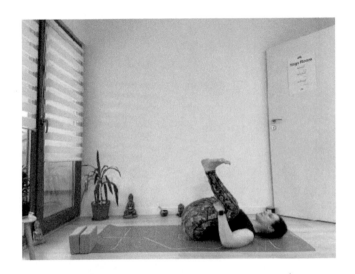

Happy Baby With Back Knee Hold

+ If you can't reach the soles of the feet without bringing the shoulders or head up, try using a yoga strap for each foot.

+ Another option is to grab the back of the knees, calves, or ankles, and you still get all the benefits.

+ If you feel discomfort in your spine area because the floor is too hard against your back, try using a folded blanket under your backside.

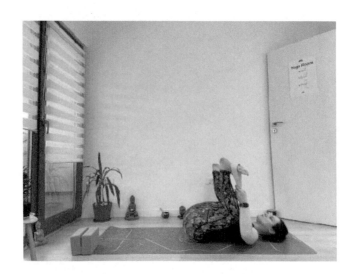

Happy Baby With Yoga Straps

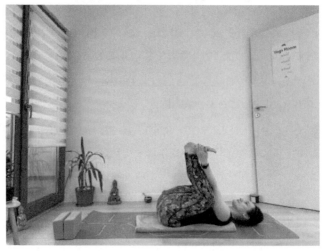

Happy Baby With Blanket

EAD TO KNEE POSE

JANUSIRSASANA

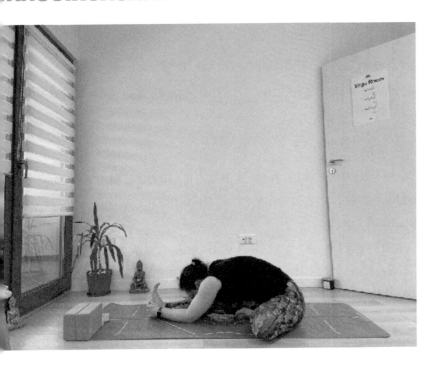

Benefits

- This pose helps soothe the nervous system, which reduces anxiety, stress, fatigue, headaches, and even mild depression
- Stretches and strengthens the lower back, groins, hamstrings, calves, and shoulders
- Increases the blood flow to the spinal nerves, colon, liver, and kidneys
- It tones the abdominal organs, which helps with digestion
- Also helps relieve menstrual and menopause discomfort and pair

How to

1. Start from sitting with both legs in front of you (Dandasana). Tilt your pelvis anteriorly and try to remove some of the "flesh" from your buttocks.
2. Bend your right knee and bring your sole to the inside of your left thigh. Rest the right knee on the mat, opening the right hip and pointing it to the side.
3. Try to keep both hips in line and facing forward. The left leg is straight, and the toes are flexed towards your chest; the back of the knees is on the mat.
4. Keep the torso upright and then slowly go down, leading with the chest and hinging from the hips. Try to bring the forehead towards the knee and rest the chest on your thigh. Make your spine long; try not to curve your back too much. Place both arms on the mat, one on each side of the left leg, being careful to keep your armpits on the same line. If you want, place your hands on the sole of the left foot.

5. Hold this pose for a few breaths, and then slowly come up and change your legs, repeating everything on the other side.

Variations

✦ If you have difficulty reaching your foot, you can use the yoga strap (belt) on the middle of your straight leg's sole and pull the ends of the strap to bring your chest closer to your thigh without curving your lower and upper back too much. You don't need to go all the way down; if that makes you lose your form, just push your chest a little bit forward with the help of the strap, letting the muscles stretch.

✦ Use a yoga block or a folded blanket under the bent knee if it's too difficult to keep it down on the mat.

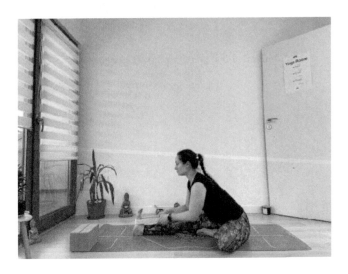

Head To Knee With Yoga Strap

✦ Elevate your hips with a block if it's too difficult to bend forward.

✦ If you tend to overextend your knee when straight, place a rolled-up blanket under it for more support. If you experience pain in the hip of the bent knee, try to bring your knee a little towards the front instead of the side.

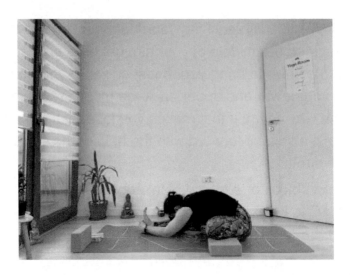

Head To Knee With Yoga Block

THREE-LIMB INTENSE STRETCH POSE

TRIANG MUKHAIKAPADA PASCHIMOTTANASANA

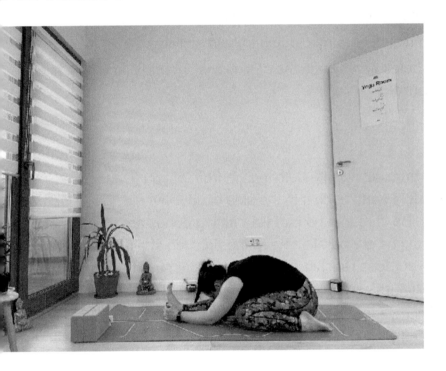

Benefits

- Improves the functioning of the liver, kidneys, and colon, like all the forward bend poses
- Gives the spine, hamstrings, and calves a good stretch
- Helps with menstrual and menopause discomfort
- It is recommended for people who suffer from flat feet and dropped arches
- Reduces stress, fatigue, and anxiety
- It stimulates parathyroid and thyroid activity
- Also helps with symptoms of sinusitis, infertility, and high blood pressure

How to

1. Start from sitting with both legs in front of you (Dandasana). Bend the left leg and bring it to the side of your left hip, like in Heron Pose. Be sure that both of your sitting bones are on the mat and your thighs are parallel. Keep the right leg straight and engaged, with your toes reaching towards your chest.
2. Keep your torso long and your spine upright, then slowly inhale, bringing your hands up. Start to fold, hinging from your hips, bringing your chest towards your thighs.
3. Grab the sides of your right sole, reaching from your forehead to your knee or shin. Push your left hip to the mat and keep your right leg engaged.
4. Bring your elbows to the side of your right leg on the mat. And relax your chest on the right thigh.

5. Hold the pose for a couple of breaths, then switch sides.

Variations

+ If you can't reach your foot, use a yoga strap around the middle of the sole. And use the ends of the strap to bring your chest closer to your thighs.
+ You can also use a yoga block under your sitting bones to help you reach the foot.
+ If your straight knee is hurting, you can place a folded blanket under it for more support. Or you can keep a slight bend in the knee to reach your chest towards your thigh.

Precautions

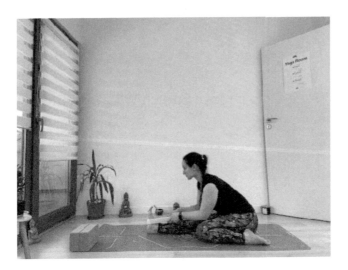

Three-Limb Intense Stretch With Yoga Strap

- ✦ It's important to take precautions when getting into the pose if you have had any surgery in the spine, hip, knee, or ankle areas.
- ✦ Take extra care when entering the pose if you have digestive issues, migraines, high blood pressure, or heart problems. Consult with your physician before trying it. And it's better to avoid it if you are pregnant.

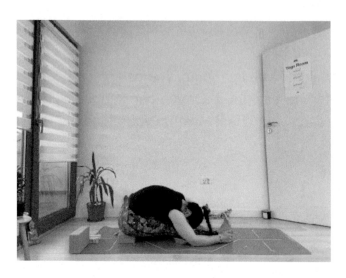

Three-Limb Intense Stretch With Yoga Block

EXTENDED HAND TO BIG TOE POSE

UTTHITA HASTA PADANGUSTASANA

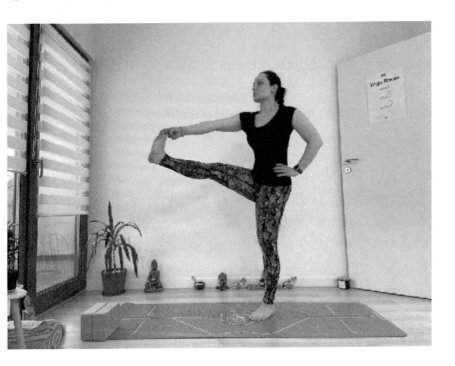

Benefits

- This pose challenges and improves not only your physical balance but also your mental one
- Stretches the hamstring of the extended leg and stabilizes the hip joint of the standing leg
- Strengthens the entire spine, shoulders, thighs, knees, calves, and ankles
- Stimulates the mind, building focus and willpower. Also cultivates poise
- Helps us improve your balance and stability

How to

1. Start from standing (Tadasana), feet shoulder width apart. Switch your weight to your left leg and slowly bring your right knee towards your chest. Keep your pelvis in a neutral position.
2. Reach inside the right leg and grab the big toe with your index and middle fingers. Bring the other hand to your hip.
3. Slowly straighten the leg, but be careful not to curve your spine. Flex your toes towards your torso while the leg is straight and pointing towards the front.
4. Keep both your hipbones in line; don't let the hip of the raised leg come up. Lift your torso upright and anteriorly tilt your pelvis so you get a better hamstring stretch. Let the natural curve of your lower back set in.
5. Keep the pose for a few breaths, then slowly release the toe and bring the knee back to your chest, then down on the mat. Shift your weight to the right leg and do the pose on the other side.

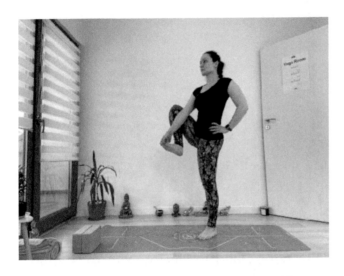

Extended Hand To Big Toe With Bent Knee

Variations

+ If your back rounds up when straightening the leg, you should keep the knee bent and hold the knee with both hands while maintaining a long spine.

+ Another variation is to use a strap around the middle of your sole and hold the ends with both hands. Slowly straighten your leg and hold it as parallel to the mat as you can. For extra help with your balance, you can use a wall or chair.

Precautions

+ Be extra careful if you have any hip or lower back issues; consult with your physician before attempting.

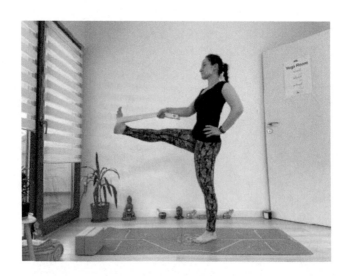

Extended Hand To Big Toe With Yoga Strap

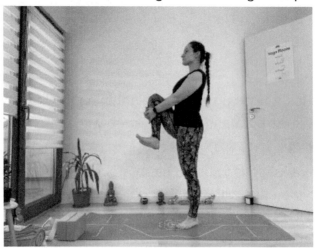

Extended Hand To Big Toe With Knee Hold

RESTING POSE

SHAVASANA

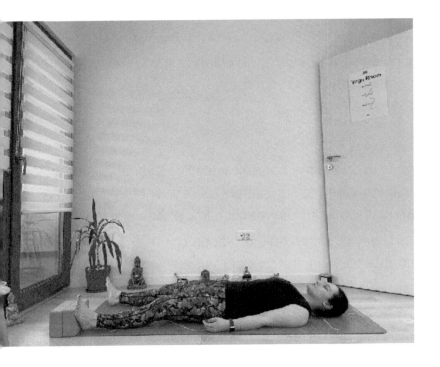

Benefits

- This pose is done after the yoga session. And it helps the body relax and rest.
- It rejuvenates and replenishes the body, giving it space and time for the benefits of the practice to sink in and promote deep healing
- Reduces anxiety and lowers blood pressure, relaxing the heart
- Helps increase your energy levels, giving your body an energy boost and increasing productivity

How to

1. This pose is one of the hardest ones I've ever encountered. Because you need to completely relax your body and mind. And if you are just a little bit like me, you know that is extremely difficult
2. We start by lying down on the mat on our backs. Find a comfortable position, but try not to use any pillows or cushions.
3. Legs are comfortably spread apart and relaxed. The toes are facing sideways and are also relaxed.
4. The arms are alongside your body and slightly apart. Palms are facing up and opened. Remember to relax them as well.
5. Now close your eyes and breathe slowly but deeply. Relax every part of the body with every exhalation.
6. Start to slowly focus on yourself and your body, letting go of all the tasks and thoughts (stuff you forgot to do; overthinking).

7. Let it all go! Be present in that moment with yourself, completely relax, and surrender. Be careful not to doze off (it happens sometimes).

8. After 10 minutes or more, depending on how much time you have, slowly start to pay attention to your breath. Then slowly wiggle your fingers and toes and slowly roll to one side, keeping your eyes closed. Stay here for one or two breaths.

9. Then gently make your way to a comfortable sitting position. Take a few deep breaths, and you can bring your palms together in front of your heart if you like. Then slowly open your eyes and begin your day with a smile.

FINAL WORDS

After doing all 18 poses, I strongly recommend taking a Shvasana (resting pose). Helps sink in all the benefits of the practice and calm the mind and body.

You can mix up the poses as you like, so you can make your own yoga flow and have fun!

You can choose your favorite poses and make your own morning routine, so you can start your day with a smile and a wonderful overall feeling. Or select easier ones for an evening routine to prepare you for a good night's sleep.

And remember, yoga isn't all about the "perfect pose", it's more about how it feels in your own body.

I sure hope these 18 yoga poses that I suggested helped you win the battle against tight hamstring muscles and back pain!

For more yoga flows and practice you can also check my website and social media

Site: www.yogawithmadalina.com

Email: contact@yogawithmadalina.com

Printed in Great Britain
by Amazon

27594163R00050